Gout Cure

Your Ultimate and Comprehensive Guide in Treating Gout Permanently

by Tammi Diamond

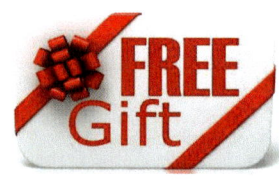

Want Priority Access to FREE eBooks Additional Materials for this Book?

As we release NEW eBooks, we offer them for FREE for a limited time. You will be the FIRST one to know when they are FREE. Join 1000's of insiders who are getting access to FREE Kindle book promotions weekly.

Click HERE for FREE additional material and FREE eBooks-
www.rictamilypublishing.com

TABLE OF CONTENTS

Introduction

Gout Defined

Causes

Symptoms

Diagnosis

Effects

Gout and its Association to Rheumatoid Arthritis

Gout and its Association to other Metabolic Syndrome

Treatment

Low-Purine Diet

Prevention

Conclusion

Review Link

Our Other Books

Dedication

Disclaimer

INTRODUCTION

I want to thank you and congratulate you for downloading the book, "**Gout Cure: Your Ultimate and Comprehensive Guide in Treating Gout**".

This book contains proven steps and strategies to understand gout and its effect and how to cure it. We will talk about its symptoms, causes and its effects. We will also talk about its association with other medical conditions. At the end of the book, we will talk about how you can treat gout symptoms and how to manage an attack and also prevention of further uric acid build up in the body. So turn the page with me and let us start learning.

Inside this book, you will learn the following things about Gout, to wit;

1. We will define comprehensively "What is Gout?" for you;
2. We will share with you the causes of Gout;
3. Likewise its Symptoms so we could easily identify it in our daily lives;
4. We will share with you diagnosis of the illness;
5. Also how it will affect our lives;
6. We will also study this illness and its association Rheumatism Arthritis;
7. And also its association with other metabolic syndrome;
8. Of course, as the title entails, its treatment, prevention and diet.

Thanks again for downloading this book, we hope you enjoy it!

CHAPTER I: Gout Defined

Gout is an inflammatory type of arthritis. It is characterized by severe pain, tenderness and swelling of the affected part. It often affects the big toe, that's about half of the cases of gout, however, it also affects the other parts of the body such as joints and some muscles.

Disease of the Kings

It is caused by the excess uric acid in the blood that gets accumulated in the joints of the body forming crystals. Uric acid comes from purine rich food such as meat, poultry and fatty fish. Gout could be traced in the olden times and often referred to as the "disease of the kings." Why? Because during those times there are many foods that only those who are in the higher level of society can afford. Chocolate is one example, some ale and meats are also consumed largely on banquets.

King Henry VIII of England is probably the most popular king to have suffered from gout. He was always depicted in pictures or paintings as someone holding a chunk of meat in one hand and a drink on the other. He was also obese which increases the risk of having gout.

Stages of Gout

There are said to be four stages of gout, which are Asymptomatic, Acute, Interval and Chronic Tophaceous. The first stage, asymptomatic is characterized by increased levels of uric acid in blood, however, there is no other symptoms, such as pain or swelling present in the patient. The Acute gout stage is characterized by intense pain which is brought about by the uric acid deposits. It can last for days, but will subside even without treatment. The interval stage is the period between attacks. In this stage, there are no symptoms experienced, like the asymptomatic stage, the uric acid level is still elevated and the chances of having a following attack are at a much higher risk. The chronic tophaceous gout is developed over a long period of time. In this stage tophi may have already developed into skin and in soft tissues.

Tophi is a mass of uric acid crystals. It forms in the skin and around the joints or on the tips of the fingers as nodes. It is considered to be a manifestation of gout in of the advanced stage. Although it usually forms around the joints, it may form just about anywhere in the body. It is also sometimes referred to as chalkstones because of its white, chalk-like appearance.

CHAPTER II: Causes

The initial cause of gout and gout attack is the elevated levels of uric acid in blood which is called hyperurecemia. Uric acid is actually a waste product of broken down chemicals in our cells called purine. Purine is obtained from food such as meat, poultry and fatty fish. That is why a low-purine diet is encouraged in people who has gout.

Aside from the dietary causes of gout, there are also some other factors affecting the risk of having gout. It could also be affected by kidney function, some metabolic syndrome and heredity.

Kidney under Excretion

Urate, the salts of uric acid are excreted by the kidney, under excretion of urate causes uric acid to stay in the blood, thus, elevating its level. When this happens, uric acid, which actually looks like tiny needles under the microscope, accumulates in the joints which causes gout attack to happen.

Metabolic Syndrome

Obesity, insulin resistance and hypertension increase the rate of the risk of having gout. It is said that the body mass has a direct relationship with the occurrence of gout. This will be further discussed in chapter vii of this eBook.

Genetics

There are rare cases where gout is hereditary. There are some genes that can be passed on from the parent to the offspring like in rare genetic disorders involving the kidney. However, this is only a small chance of having and there is only very little documentation on the occurrence of these conditions. Familial lifestyle, however, is more known to have an effect on the offspring of a parent who has gout as lifestyle could also be inherited and passed on, therefore, making gout indirectly hereditary. Children of parents who has gout could already take precautionary measures by watching what they eat, watching their alcohol intake and making exercise a habit.

Triggers

Aside from the causes listed above, the actual gout attack is triggered by some factors. This includes stress at work, accidents, strenuous work or workouts and major operations. While there is no actual study linking these triggers directly to the disease, attacks are preceded by one or two of these factors.

CHAPTER III: Symptoms

Gout is generally characterized with gout attacks with intense pain that happens mostly during the night. The intense pain is usually localized to a certain area, most of the time, in the big toe, but could also be in the large joints of the body such as ankles, knees, wrist and elbows. The area affected could mostly be swollen, red and tender. Heat, which is feels almost like a fever, could also result from the debilitating pain.

While initial symptom of gout is evident with a high level of uric acid in blood. Symptoms of gout differ from one stage to another.

During the early stage of gout, it could be asymptomatic, meaning there is no physical manifestation of the disease aside from a high level of uric acid in blood. This is also true with the interval stage, which is the stage between the gout attacks.

It is during the acute stage that the intense pain is initially felt combined with the swelling and tenderness of the affected area. During this stage, the pain could go away for hours to two days and no medication is even required, but precautions should already be taken to avoid the next attack.

During the advance stage of gout, which is developed over a long period of time, usually an average of ten years, tophi are mostly present in patients. These are nodes of mass of uric acid crystals. It is usually developed around the joints, at the tips of the fingers and at the tip of the elbow and knees. However, it could also be formed anywhere like in the skin and around the ears. Also, during the advance stage, the pain could get more intense and could take longer to subside. In some cases, the pain could last to up to two weeks.

CHAPTER IV: Diagnosis

Gout has classic symptoms that in some cases a diagnostic exam is not anymore needed to diagnose a person with gout. This is usually in the case of Podagra, which is characterized with the pain in the big toe. However, in some cases, a test should be performed in order to rule other diseases out as gout may be mistaken as other diseases such as in cases of rheumatoid arthritis and, if there is a presence of tophi in the skin, it could be mistaken as basal cell carcinoma.

The following are the basic diagnostic exam being performed on patients believed to have gout.

Identification of Urate crystals in Synovial Fluid

The synovial fluid is the fluid found in between the joints. It functions as a kind of a lubricant between the bones and the cartilage. Testing the synovial fluid for traces of urate crystals in it is the definitive method of diagnosing gout. Finding a needle-like urate crystals under a polarized microscope is a positive test. This is a very hard test to perform and only done with laboratory personnel who are specially trained to perform this test.

Blood Testing

> **Chemistry** - In males, above a plasma urate level of 420 umol/l, and in females, above a plasma urate level of 360 umol/l is a positive result, also a classic characteristic of gout.
>
> **Hematology** - Increase in white blood cells in the absence of infection is a positive test and is indicative of gout.
>
> **Renal Function** - very low creatinine clearance is associated with gout. In this case the kidney may under excrete the uric acid in the blood resulting in uric acid build-up.

CHAPTER V: Effects

As what is mentioned at the start of this book, gout is a very serious disease. In fact, it is very serious that its effects could be life-altering. The pain which is associated with this disease is notorious with rendering the patient immobile for days, most of the time missing a lot of time from work and from their family.

After the initial attack, the patient becomes aware that a second attack may come and this is the time when a person becomes conscious of what he eats and the activities that he does. They may find themselves limited from eating or doing many things. This sudden change does not only affect his day-to-day activities, but could also affect his overall outlook in life.

Change in mobility

People who had an experience having their first gout attacks are more conscious in doing many things that includes long walks or climb. They become worried that they may not be able to do things on their own when an attack caught up to them. They become worried that they may suffer an attack while doing things like driving. These affect people greatly and a huge change may be noticed in patients.

Dietary changes

After the initial attack, a gout patient is advised to go on a low purine diet. To some people who has not experienced dieting before, this could be a very difficult time and could take a long while of getting used to. In some cases, drastic diet change results in a form of a state of shock, physical manifestations such as the hands trembling may be noticed. Also a change in mood is quite noticeable.

Lifestyle

A person who has gout may find himself not only limited to what he can do physically and what he can eat, but also he may find himself not being able to enjoy some of the things he enjoys before he was diagnosed with the disease. People who likes going out to party and drink once in a while will find themselves not being able to do it anymore or that they have to control themselves to only drink a little or party a little when they have this disease.

Outlook
Because of the gout a person may find themselves insufficient, especially when they have already started missing work because of the pain. Some highly driven individuals may find themselves taken aback by the disease and therefore may lose their confidence in the process. The pain also mostly makes a person more sensitive to their feelings and when their joints or bodies become deformed because of the presence of tophi, they may become ashamed of their appearance and may prefer to stay home instead of going out to exercise.

CHAPTER VI: Gout and its Association to Rheumatoid Arthritis

Since gout is a form of arthritis, it is often mistaken as one of its other forms, the Rheumatoid Arthritis. They have almost very similar signs and symptoms. Yes, there is that classic pain, swelling, redness and tenderness. But that's just it. Gout is a kind of inflammatory types of arthritis caused by high levels of uric acid while Rheumatoid Arthritis is an autoimmune disease, which attacks the persons' own muscles, and is of unknown cause. The cause, the cure and other characteristic are entirely different between the two.

So how do you know which one you got?

Here is a chart comparison between the two which clearly shows their great difference.

	Gout	**Rheumatoid Arthritis**
Signs and Symtoms	Intense pain, redness, swelling, tenderness, formation of tophi	Intense pain, redness, swelling, tenderness
Area affected	Big Toe, joints, other body parts	Joints, other body parts
Cause	Accumulation of uric acid in blood and joints	Unknown
Type of disease	Metabolic	Autoimmune
Diagnosis	Uric acid level	Inflammatory markers
Gender	Usually males	Usually Females
Treatment	NSAIDs, Colchicine, steroids, Urocosuric	NSAIDs, Steroids, DMARDs (Methotrexate)

CHAPTER VII: Gout and its Association to other Metabolic Syndrome

Metabolic syndrome is a group of conditions that occur as a risk factor of heart disease, diabetes and stroke. These conditions include high blood pressure, obesity, high blood sugar level, abdominal fat and increased cholesterol level.

Not all of the conditions are always present in one patient, however, the presence of one condition is enough indication of a disease.

Although indirectly, metabolic syndrome has always been associated with gout. If a person has gout, there is a big chance that he also has metabolic syndrome. This is also the reason why people with gout is at high risk of having heart diseases, stroke and diabetes.

The association of gout and the metabolic syndrome may be attributed to its cause. Both gout and the conditions in the metabolic syndrome all comes from the food we eat and the lifestyle that we have. Often, people who are obese and are inactive are those who are affected with these diseases.

Both gout and the metabolic syndrome are also associated with insulin resistance and kidney failure. A decrease in kidney function may lead to under excretion of waste material in the blood, which may cause some of these conditions as well as gout.

CHAPTER VIII: Treatment

Treatment for gout differs depending on the symptoms and the frequency of attacks. Basically, drugs that are readily available in your local drugstores aims to treat and ease the intense pain. When the primary symptoms have been treated, doctors will prescribe medicine to prevent future attacks. There are many options about the kind of treatments that you may choose from.

Acute Gout Attack Treatment

Nonsteroidal Anti-inflammatory Drugs (NSAIDs)

NSAIDs are probably the most prescribed drugs for gout sufferers. It is the most effective drug for acute gout attacks. It can make a person better within hours of the attack. However, it may not be used by persons who have gastrointestinal problems.

Colchicine

Colchicine is an alternative drug or maybe taken with NSAIDs. It is also an effective treatment for acute gout attacks. However, colchicine takes long time to effect compared with NSAIDs. It is said to be most effective when taken at 12 hours after the attack.

Steroid

Steroids, mainly, corticosteroids are given mostly to alleviate intense pain. It is very effective and could act almost instantaneously. It could be injected straight into the affected joint or given intravenously in patients who are confined in the hospital.

Preventive Medications

In cases when people would have repeat episodes of attacks, doctors would prescribe xanthine oxidase inhibitor drugs. These drugs act as uric acid production blocker. Most of the time allopurinol or febuxostat are prescribed. However, there are times when contraindication with this drug may occur. In cases when there is contraindication with xanthine inhibitor drugs of if the uric acid is not too high, urocosics drugs may be given.

Natural Gout Treatment

Cold Compress

In cases when there is an acute gout attack and intense pain may be experienced, applying cold compress may help ease some of the pain if applied directly to the affected area. You may put an ice bag directly over it or a small block of ice wrapped in a towel.

Increase water intake

Water may help in flushing excess uric acid in blood. It is best to keep your body hydrated to prevent further attacks.

CHAPTER IX: Low-Purine Diet

As what is discussed earlier, uric acids, which cause gout is a product of breaking down purine which we get from the food we eat. This is mainly the reason why doctors suggest a drastic dietary change in people diagnosed with gout. They are advised to switch to a low-purine diet. What is a low purine diet?

It just basically means limiting your intake of food rich in purine. There are many low-purine diet plans that you can find in the Internet. You can practically choose what will best suit you. In this chapter, we will give you an overview of what you can eat and what to avoid in a low-purine diet.

What to avoid?

There are foods that you can enjoy when you are on a low-purine diet and there are foods that you can have a little of in a controlled manner. But there are those that are a total no-no. These foods are found to make your gout worsen and may cause irreversible damage to your body. These are notorious and are better left out of your diet or endure a painful fate. I know, we all do not want that. So, here is a list of what to avoid.

Meat Group

- Bacon, veal and venison, liver, processed meat

Seafood Group

- Anchovies, sardines, codfish, mussels, scallops, trout, herring

Sauces

- Gravy

Drinks

- Beer, soft drinks (because of fructose content)

What can be taken in moderation?

Meat group

- Chicken, beef, or pork

Seafood Group

- Crab, lobster, oysters and shrimp

Dairy group
    - Eggs

Drinks
    - Liquor or wine, coffee

What can be enjoyed?

Dairy group
    - Low-fat and fat-free dairy products, such as cheese and yogurt

Carbohydrates-rich foods
    - Rice, noodles, pasta and potatoes

Fruit and Vegetable Group
    - All of them

Drinks
    - Plenty of fluids, such as water or fruit juice

CHAPTER X: Prevention

Although there are drugs that are readily available in your local drugstores for gout attacks, these only targets to ease the intense pain and other symptoms of gout. It does not actually prevent you from having another attack. You may use uric acid formation blockers, but there are already uric acids in your blood to start with. It's because we can only do so much.

You will be surprised to know that prevention of gout and gout attack are mostly practical in nature. These are little things that we can practice and live by to prevent a debilitating attack from happening. So, what are these things that we can do, you may ask. These are just simple everyday things, here is a list of ways how we can prevent gout and gout attack from happening.

Mind your diet

If you have a family history of gout, you may start early and keep your diet in check. You may still eat everything but some food should already be taken in moderation. On the other hand, if you are already diagnosed with gout, you have to follow a strict diet. Avoid foods that are very rich in purine, some food may be taken in moderation, but those foods that are blacklisted should not be included in your diet in any way.

Always take time to drink water as it may help to flush the toxins out of your body. It will not only flush out excess uric acids, it will also flush out cholesterol and excess sugar that causes other metabolic diseases which is a risk factor of gout.

Exercise and lose weight

Make it a habit to move your body. It is not an excuse that you do not have time to work out or to exercise. There are simple ways how we can move our bodies. You may take the stairs instead of taking the elevator, for example, or walking instead of driving to a store near your house. It does not have to always be a strenuous exercise. You can do anything that is enough to keep your blood flowing.

You will lose weight gradually. As we have discussed earlier, obesity is a risk factor of gout as well as the metabolic syndrome. Gradually losing weight could improve your health greatly. Take note, however, that it has to be gradual, otherwise, your body may be in shock if you lose weight drastically.

Got to have a regular check-up

Visiting your doctor and following your doctor's advice religiously will help you to prevent the occurrence of gout. Also, having a regular blood test could check if the medications you are taking are taking effect. If you will not have a regular check-up, monitoring of your health progress will be hard and detection of complications could be very late.

Conclusion

Gout is not a rare disease. It could happen to anyone. It could strike an attack while you are sleeping. It could also happen even if you are young. There are many studies that have been made for the treatment of gout and there are people who are successful in maintaining their health. They were able to bounce back after an attack and they were able to get a hold of their lives again.

It is better said than done, I know. But, it is up to you how to choose. This eBook is just a guide to help you manage your disease. The work will all be done by you. I guess the most important thing to remember here is gout can be prevented. The best thing for you to do is to make the first steps of prevention. Consult your doctors and live an active and healthy life.

Review Link

If you enjoyed this book, we would really appreciate it if you could leave us a positive REVIEW?

P.S. **You can CLICK HERE to go directly to the book page** and leave your review and/or purchase our other books above. Alternatively, you can copy and paste this address into your browser --- http://amzn.to/1wCj3OE

Our Other Books

THE AD: A Mal-Order Bride Romance Series

ANTI-CANCER DIET: The Ultimate Guide in Fighting Cancer, Lowering Cancer Risk and Achieving Optimum Health

10 THINGS YOU NEED TO KNOW ABOUT EBOLA: Facts about the Virus, Symptoms, Quarantine and Prevention

ULTIMATE GUIDE TO FINANCIAL FREEDOM: Achieve Wealth, Attain Success and Manage your Debt like the Rich!

GILGAMESH: King of Immortality – An Extra Biblical Proof for the Genesis Flood

HERBAL SOAP MAKING: How to Make Homemade Herbal Soaps that Clean and Nurture the Body!

PILATES FOR BEGINNERS: The Essential Guide to Total Body Fitness, Strong Muscles and Lean Body

TEETH HEALING THROUGH OIL PULLING: The Complete Guide in Natural Oral Care through the Benefits of Oil Pulling

Dedication

To our three blessings that have made RicTamily complete and continue to grow together in His loving embrace.

Disclaimer

The information in this book is in no way intended as medical advice. This book is not meant to be used, nor should it be used, to diagnose or treat any medical condition. The author disclaims responsibility for any adverse health effects that come in combination with the use of methods and suggestions presented in the book. The publisher and author are not responsible for any health or allergy needs that may require medical supervision and are not liable for any damages or negative consequences from any treatment, action, application or preparation, to any person reading or following the information in this book.

Printed in Great Britain
by Amazon